362.175

T re

Who? Me?

A journal of 50 word thoughts on
Living with Breast Cancer

By Kathy Newitt

Bloomington, IN  Milton Keynes, UK

AuthorHouse™
1663 Liberty Drive, Suite 200
Bloomington, IN 47403
www.authorhouse.com
Phone: 1-800-839-8640

AuthorHouse™ UK Ltd.
500 Avebury Boulevard
Central Milton Keynes, MK9 2BE
www.authorhouse.co.uk
Phone: 08001974150

© 2006 Kathy Newitt. All rights reserved.

This book is a work of non-fiction. Unless otherwise noted, the author and the publisher make no explicit guarantees as to the accuracy of the information contained in this book.

No part of this book may be reproduced, stored in a retrieval system, or transmitted by any means without the written permission of the author.

First published by AuthorHouse 6/26/2006

ISBN: 1-4259-3759-4 (sc)

Printed in the United States of America
Bloomington, Indiana

This book is printed on acid-free paper.

Lyrics in thought titled TELL ME IT'S NOT TRUE is from Blood Brothers by Willy Russell published by Methuen Publishing Ltd

The affirmation in thought titled AFFIRMATION has been printed with permission from Self-Esteem and Peak Performance by Jack Canfield. Boulder, CO: Career Track, 1988.

Cover illustration by Peter Moulton
www.petermoulton.com

Dedication

For my mother who inspired my inquisitive nature

How lucky for me
That you were chosen
To be my mother

How lucky I am
To have had you
To guide me through life

What fortune I have had
To learn from gentle,
Peaceful you

Thank you for my life,
Thank you for your love,
Dear mother, dear friend

Acknowledgements

To everyone in my life who has kept me in their thoughts and prayers. Thank you.

A special thank you to my chemo buddy

CONTENTS

IN THE BEGINNING	1
SURGERY	17
CHEMOTHERAPY	25
RADIOTHERAPY	43
POST TREATMENTS	53
HAIR	59
BREASTS	77
FRIENDS	81
ANNIVERSARIES	87
GENERALLY SPEAKING	93

I AM WRITING THIS BECAUSE…

I never want to forget the impact of this episode in my life. I want to remember how brave I've been. It hasn't been an easy ride, but I've learned such a lot along the way. I've weathered a severe storm; I want to hang on to this proud feeling.

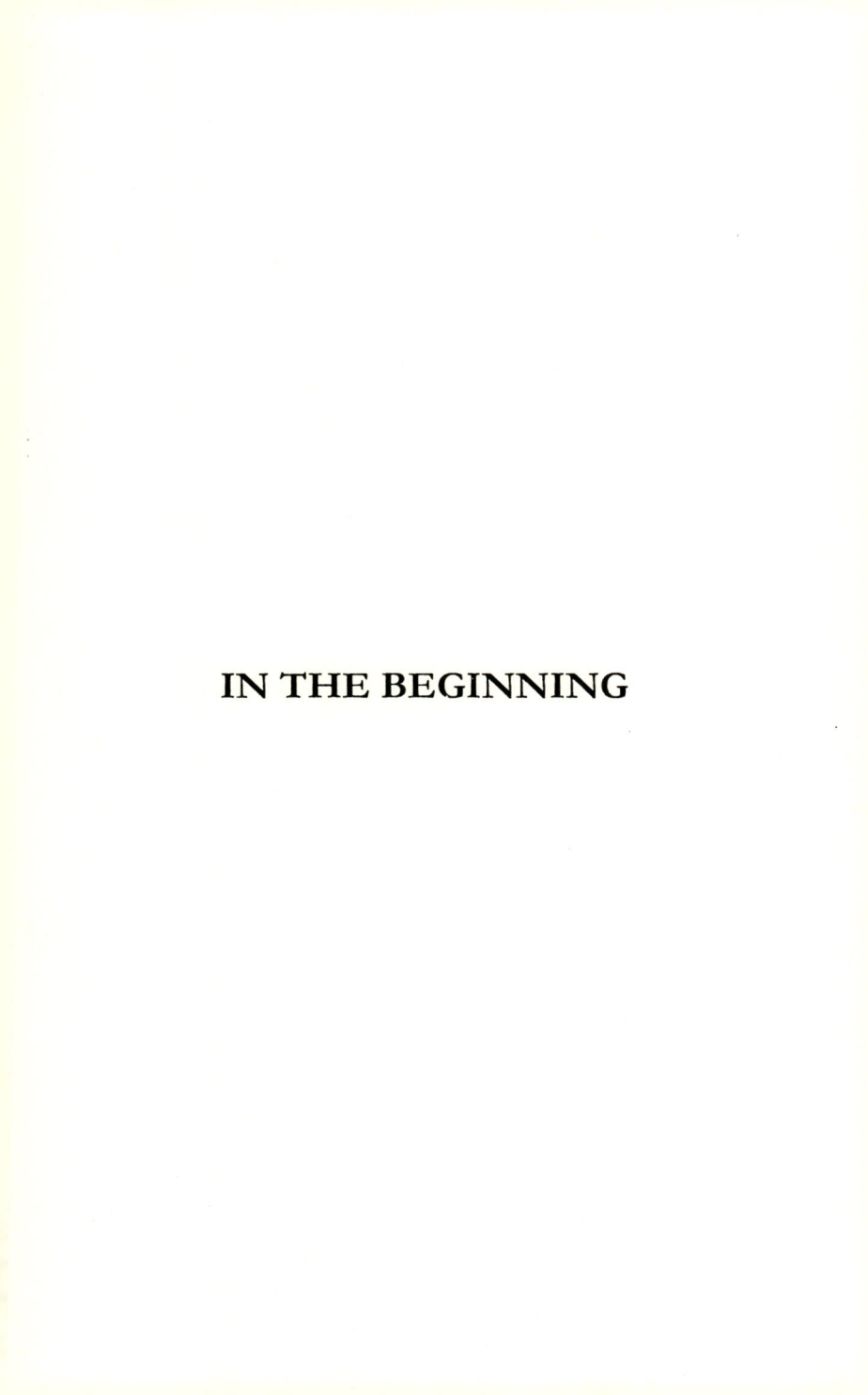

IN THE BEGINNING

THE PAUSE

I can't get used to being old enough to be having menopausal symptoms. The strangest thing I've had to get used to is excess weight. I have been slender all of my life, until now. And with the weight comes ample breasts, complete with cleavage. That's something I never expected!

HOT FLUSHES

'Did you know the radiator is set very low', my husband asks.
'Yes. And the patio door is open. And there's a pile of my clothes on the floor beside me. I'm hot.'

I no longer complain about hot flushes. Without hot flushes I would not have discovered my lump.

KITCHEN WINDOW

Every time I open that kitchen window now the *déjà vu* creeps over me.
I'm standing facing the grey tile by the kettle, silently congratulating myself for being in such good health at age 50. I open the window and pat myself down from a flush and feel the lump…

FIRST REACTION

Just when I'm getting used to having ample breasts I find a lump; bugger. My mind starts to roll. No, feel again, and again; doctor, clinic, mammogram, biopsy, sad family, widower, motherless children, not me, not ready; plan funeral, think positive thoughts …
All these thoughts within first 60 seconds.

PLEASE NOT ME

I am taking my daily routine walk. My mind is not settled. I am looking towards the beautiful green fields laid out before me but I do not see them. That lump is invading my thoughts. *It won't be cancer. Don't worry unnecessarily. Be optimistic. Not me. Please not me.*

I'M GOING TO MAKE A DOCTOR'S APPOINTMENT

This is how I tell my husband I have found a lump.
I choose to go alone but he's home when I return from my appointment.
'She felt my lump. She's making me a clinic appointment.'
I'm weeping now.
'I don't want the medical profession to take over my life.'

LACK OF CONCENTRATION

I continue my various weekly activities, acting on the outside as if life is normal. I haven't told everyone about my lump. I converse, engage in idle chat. I think I respond appropriately, but all the while my mind is focussed on one thing only: *I have a lump.*

TALE OF WOE

I've come to tell you my tale of woe.
Oh. Is it the cats?
No. It's me.
Come in, sit down; tell me.
I've found a lump in my breast. I have an appointment at the clinic for a biopsy next week.
Oh Kathy. I'm sorry. What can I do?

WHAT SHOULD I EXPECT?

I ring the clinic prior to my visit. Knowing what to expect removes some of the anxiety.

'A consultant will examine you and perform a fine needle aspiration. Then you'll have a mammogram and possibly a needle biopsy. There may be some discomfort. Diagnosis should reach you in five days.'

CLINIC

Rainy day; struggle to park. Book in; wait.
First consultant: fine needle aspiration.
'It could be nothing, try not to panic.'
I liked that doctor.
Different building. Mammogram.
Wait   Wait   Wait
Needle biopsy.
'Cup of tea?'
'No thanks'
'I'll be surprised if that's not cancer.'
I didn't like that radiologist.

STUNNED

I was prepared for the possibility of cancer but I wasn't told the radiologist would be hazarding a guess at my diagnosis before samples were studied. I felt he was tactless; I never wanted to see him again. I was upset; stunned. I didn't expect that at my initial appointment.

DIAGNOSIS

'Last week you came to see us and had a number of tests …'
'Yes, get on with it.'
'The biopsy did come back positive for cancer …'
'Kathy has cancer. How weird is that? I have cancer …'
'Do you have any questions?'
'Yes, is the …'
'I have cancer, cancer, cancer, CANCER!'

IN A FUZZ

I'm familiar with the words: *breast lump, cancer, statistic, treatment regime.*
But they're not supposed to apply to me. I listen with fuzzy ears and want to shout,
'WHO? ME? ARE YOU TALKING ABOUT *ME*?'
These things happen to other people, not to me.

Oh dear, wrong again. *Damn* it!

BRRRRRRRRRRRRRRNG
Wake up call

What's that lump in my breast? Cancer? No bloody way. Where the hell did that come from? If no one can tell me, how on earth am I supposed to prevent it from recurring? Why me? Why *bloody* me?

It's out of my control. Time to take up the challenge.

UNIVERSAL TEACHER'S REVIEW BOARD

'She's very good at giving.'
'Yes, but lacks ability to receive.'
'What shall we do to remedy that?'
'She needs a tough lesson. She needs to learn the lesson so there will be no turning back.'
'Not another one.'
'I'm afraid so.'
'Cancer it is then. Next case.'

NUMB

I am ironing; the phone rings.
'Hello?'
'Hi Kathy, it's Roger. How are you?'
'Well, I can't say I'm fine to be honest, (*pause*) I've been diagnosed with breast cancer.'
'Oh dear. (*silence*) How are you feeling about that?'
'I don't know really. Numb. I don't actually believe it …'

INSULTED

I find this cancer diagnosis quite an insult. I've been conscious of my health for years and have taken positive steps towards healthy living. Perfect I'm not, but really, why me? What have I done wrong? Is it related to diet? Somebody tell me so I can put it right.

I DON'T FEEL A THING

How can I have cancer when I feel so fit? I have no physical symptoms, bar a painless, invisible lump. How can that small mass within my breast be so potentially devastating when I feel so fit? Its physical impact is only a concept. Its emotional impact is very real.

I WANT

I want to be an oncologist, a haematologist, a radiologist, a breast surgeon, a toxicologist. I want to understand every minute detail of what is going on with my body. I want to know what questions to ask and how to understand the answers. Is that too much to ask?

FAILING THAT

Failing realising above wants, I settle with doing my own research, beginning with the internet. I formulate a comprehensive set of questions before meeting my doctors. I don't need to ask all questions, but having made the list helped me to listen and better comprehend what I was being told.

HUNGRY FOR INFO

I continue my research. The more I know, the better I feel. I borrow books, buy books, talk with friends, read magazines, search internet. I munch my way through piles of information and end up feeling like *The Very Hungry Caterpillar* – full to overflowing.
Time to put the books aside.

PRAYERS

I've grown up with prayer, being of a Catholic background, but it was just a concept until cancer entered my life. I experienced the effect when I shared my news. The response was notification of prayers from family, friends, friend's friends … and so it went. And so I coped.

FEAR NOT

Fear not? You think?! I tried to kid myself I was fearless when confronted with confirmation of my cancer diagnosis. I thought fear would sap my energy. I thought fear was a negative feeling. But when I let myself feel the fear I began to take charge and move forward.

MY NEW JOB

My new job is to look after me, to rest, nurture myself; make sure I'm as fit as possible to endure upcoming aggressive therapies. Maintain healthy diet, stay focussed and positive. This is what my family and friends are encouraging me to do and I'm going to follow their advice

TREATMENT PLAN

The cancerous lump in my left breast will be surgically removed. Chemotherapy begins six to eight weeks after surgery, taking up to eighteen weeks. Three weeks after chemotherapy finishes there follows fifteen consecutive radiotherapy sessions, bar weekends.
Seven months of my precious life gone by and treatments will be finished.

THE BOYS TAKE CHARGE

'I've got it all organised. When you get out of hospital I'll do the cooking and Joe will do the shopping and vacuuming.'
'What's dad's job?'
'He's project manager!'
Dad took on the job of laundry.
My, they were busy!
How lovely to rest guiltlessly whilst my boys take charge.

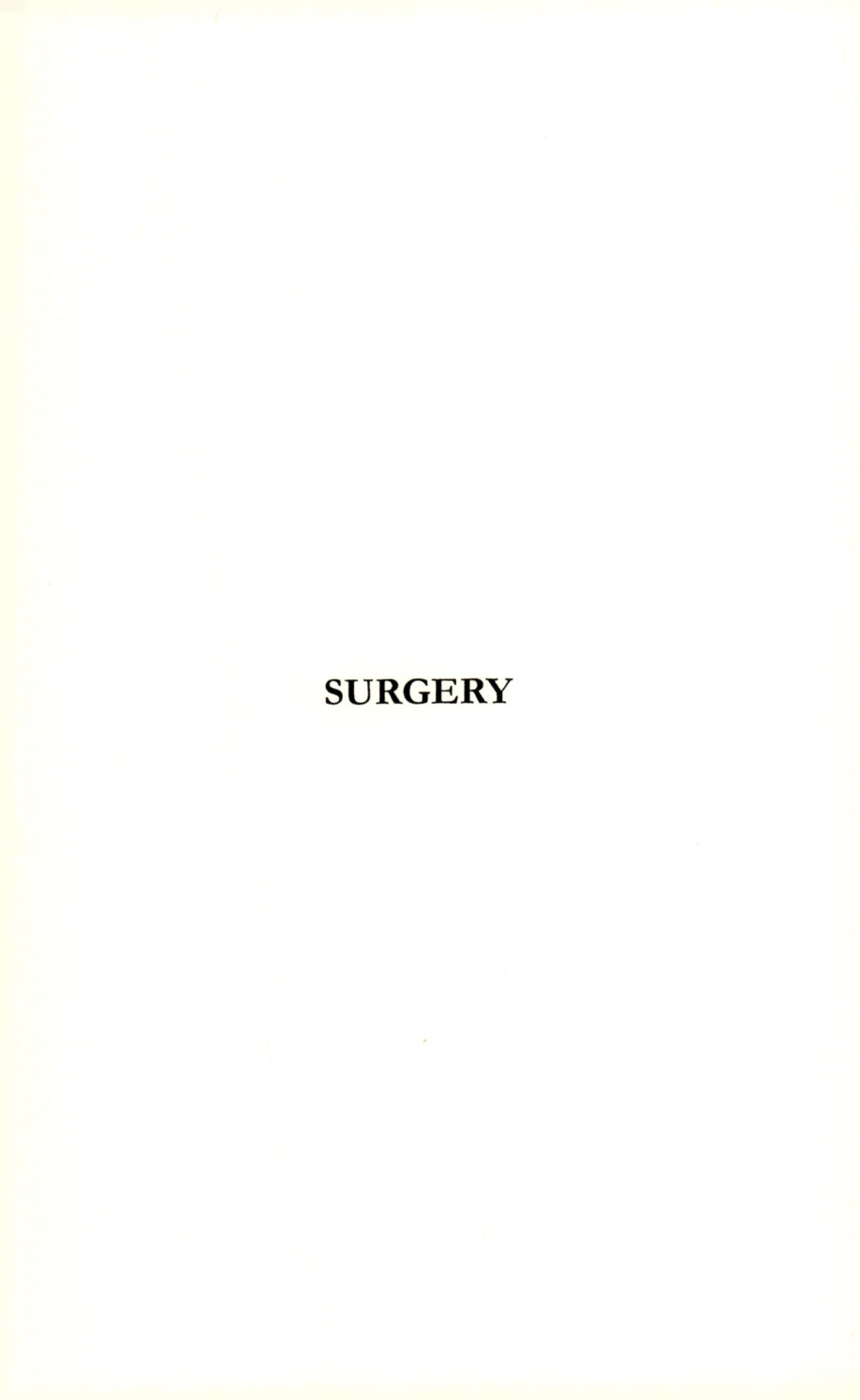

SURGERY

THE DAY HAS COME

We're due at hospital at noon. Post arrives delivering a parcel from a friend containing a beautiful crystal pendant. Good timing. There's also a brochure advertising a China tour. Browsing Mastertravel's website, my article appears; first time I'd seen it online. Good day to find it. The morning's passing pleasantly.

ARRIVAL

Don't know how I appear externally, internally I feel like a frightened rabbit. My innards are quivering, my chest is tight; my eyes are focussed determinedly ahead. I am using quite a lot of energy just preventing myself from giving way and collapsing.
I can do this. I am strong.

FIRST STOP – NUCLEAR MEDICINE

Nuclear medicine? How scary is that?! A blue dye is injected into my tumour site and I'm asked to return in a couple of hours for the 'photo session'. These images will enable the surgeon to locate the sentinel node thus preventing me from losing an unnecessary number of nodes.

PHOTO SESSION

I was told they'd take two photos. They didn't tell me each photo would take seven minutes. As I lie in the machine, arms above my head, concentrating on being still, reality hits, the tears escape. Must be true; time to face it. I do have cancer. Surgery is imminent.

SETTLING IN

Book in at noon, surgery at 6:30pm; that's a lot of hours in between. Tests, 'photo session', nurse's questions, meet the anaesthetist, order from breakfast menu. I unpack; make myself at home for my two night visit. Gown and surgical socks brought in, it must be getting near the time.

THE TIME HAS COME

I feel like I'm on ER. I watch the ceiling as the gurney is wheeled to the lift whereupon we are transported to the operating theatre. Anteroom resembles a storage cupboard. Anaesthetist inserts the needle in my hand and I gather my angels for support as I drift into oblivion.

SHAKES

…next thing I know I am being wheeled down a corridor with lots of people around me. My body is shaking uncontrollably; I can see blurred images and hear voices commenting on my shaking. Hands steady me and I wonder if I'll fall off the gurney. Suddenly, the shaking stops.

MINUTES SLOWLY TICKING BY

I don't know what's up with that clock, it's moving ever so slowly. Family have come and gone, I doze, wake, 5 minutes have passed. I sip water, doze, wake, check breast, (still there), doze, wake again; only 2am. I'm feeling very 'swimmy'. This is good stuff they've given me!

BEWARE THE CAT

I'm sent home with lymph drainage tube intact.

My cat was most interested in this device last week when the breast care nurse came to the house to explain details of my imminent hospital stay.

I keep it well hidden beneath my bathrobe. It is removed the following day - phew!

CHRISTMAS DAY

I've been home for two days. The boys are busy in the kitchen tackling Christmas dinner. I'm sitting, napping on and off. We've opened gifts in our tastefully decorated room. (I spent two weeks pre-surgery passing time decorating house.) The boys' roast turkey dinner with trimmings is a real treat.

PRACTICE WHAT YOU PREACH

Before attending the retreat at the Bristol Cancer Help Centre I watch the introductory video. I feel I'm in tune with their philosophy: positive thinking, relaxation, good nutrition … I have recommended the same to my reflexology clients. I book a place and look forward to practising what I preach.

RETREAT

I'd always wanted to go on a retreat and in my hour of need, the opportunity arose. I share five days of peaceful bliss with nine people also dealing with cancer. Serenity prevailed. Moral support abounded. I experienced wonderful food, good advice, tears and laughter. It was the perfect tonic.

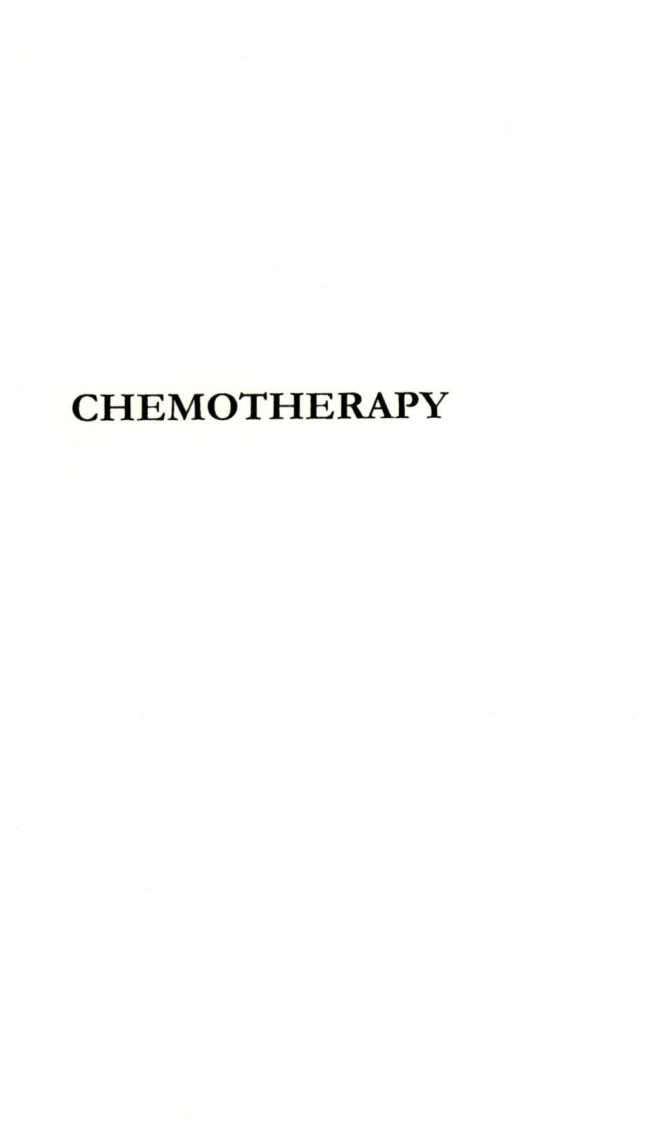

CHEMOTHERAPY

SURVIVAL RATE

All of a sudden I'm a statistic. My survival rate over 10 years is 75%. Women with similar prognosis who do have chemotherapy have a slightly higher percentage of survival than those who don't. It is truly bizarre listening to someone discuss your survival rate. The concept of mortality sharpens.

WHAT SHALL I DO?

Agreeing to chemotherapy is the most difficult decision I've ever made. Had doctor been able to say this treatment definitely prevents recurrence I would have agreed without question. Accepting chemo as a 'just in case' measure may have been the wise choice, but it was a hard pill to swallow.

PEACE OF MIND

When first faced with the dilemma of treatment choices my focus was short; I just wanted the shortest route to the end. After weeks of deliberation I was able to consider the bigger picture. Five months would soon pass. I decided chemo was my only hope for peace of mind.

NOW I'VE DECIDED...

... I see chemotherapy as a challenge. I am determined I will survive each treatment with minimal effects. I follow my healthy diet religiously, practice qigong daily, use bach flower remedies to calm my emotional state, I rest; have regular reflexology, share my woes with friends. And all to good effect.

CHEMO BUDDY

When telling one of my best friends of my decision to go ahead with chemo she asked if I would like company at the chemo sessions. Now I won't have to face the dreaded appointments alone. How blessed am I to have such a dear friend? Thank you chemo buddy.

CHEMO CAPS

Someone I am only acquainted with via an internet scrabble site made a very kind offer when I mentioned my cancer diagnosis.
'Would you like me to make you some chemo caps?'
A chemo cap is a warm crocheted skull cap. I'm fortunate to be the recipient of such kindness.

YOU HAVE TO BE NICE TO ME

A friendly banter between me and my son:
You have to be nice to me because I have cancer.
No you don't. The surgeon took it away.
Fair enough. But you still have to be nice to me because
I have chemotherapy. You can't deny that.
Oh OK. You win.

FIRST TIME

After conquering my fear of having chemotherapy I find myself sitting in the oncology waiting room happily chatting with my chemo buddy. I knew it would be a long wait, but after 2½ of hours of watching the minutes tick by I am back to square one - *feeling the fear*.

ANGELS

chemo visualisation

They're microscopic and they stream down with the moon's beams to my rescue, my little angels. They melt beneath my skin and set to, cleaning up after the cancer therapies. Some nurture good cells others eradicate bad cells. I continue healing with my team of little angels working for me.

INCREDIBLE JOURNEY

I would like to turn my cancer into an incredible journey. Microscopic me would be injected into my body carrying special cancer sensors and zappers, and at the end of the journey I would return knowing for certain I am cancer free and will remain so. Wouldn't that be incredible?

WAITING FOR ANOTHER BLOOD TEST

Today is my second blood test since starting chemotherapy. Forty minutes pass before my number comes up.
'Have you been waiting?'
'Yes'
'You don't have to wait if you're a chemo patient. You don't want to be sitting with all those germs.'
'Oh.'
That will make future visits more tolerable.

PHYSICAL vs EMOTIONAL

I'm finding being philosophical about my physical symptoms quite easy. Don't know why. Tabs for sickness, seabands for nausea, slippery elm for constipation, scarf in place of hair. So why is dealing with the emotional turmoil so much more difficult? Thank God my many supporters are available to keep me afloat.

STEROIDS

I queried the need for steroids at my pre-chemo chat with the nurse. She explained they helped quell nausea but weren't necessary for chemo's effectiveness.
Steroids made me anxious and depressed. After my third treatment I requested they be removed from all future treatments. I'd rather feel nauseous than depressed.

GOOD MEDICINE

I came to look upon my diet as my good medicine. I believe my healthy diet balanced the toxic therapies. Making sure the healthiest foods possible nurtured my body gave me back some of the control over my wellbeing that the cancer took away. Having some control kept me strong.

SYMPTOMS

I'm glad chemo didn't mess with my taste buds. My healthy diet was my salvation. Eating good food remained a pleasure. Chemo did however alter my olfactory sense. There were certain aromas that turned my stomach; fresh coffee brewing, spicy curries cooking. Fortunately these were not included in my diet.

REALITY HITS

It is only the day before each chemo treatment that it hits me how weird it is to let someone sit opposite me and pump toxins into my veins. This thought makes me feel as cold as the first drug that wends its icy path in search of cancer cells.

BOTHER!

I knew this was going to happen at some time during my chemotherapy, yet I'm totally taken aback now that is has. I received phone call today –
'Bloods too low; will have to delay until next week.'
Firsts are always the hardest and I'm feeling enormously disappointed.
Bother, bother, *bother!*

PHONE CALLS

Now it's happened once I am on tenterhooks the day before each chemo. Blood test in morning - wonder if nurse will ring to say bloods are low again. All of these little things build up to one big emotional turmoil. Sometimes I'd like life to be a little less challenging.

WELCOME TO THE CHEMO CLUB

The fifth chemo treatment was the only one that made me feel like a chemo patient. Nausea began fours hours after treatment and it hit hard. I curled up in bed with sick bowl for two days. I focussed on day three when nausea was likely to ease; and slept.

TOO FAR

The phone is ringing. I lie motionless, considering whether or not to act on my automatic response to answer.
The phone is three feet away - too far.
If I move, the nausea will return. I don't have the energy to converse anyway.
The ringing stops. Thank goodness.
Sleep returns.

MAKEUP

This morning I'm too weak to stand in front of the mirror to apply my makeup. I take makeup mirror and supplies to desktop and sit down. I'm not expecting visitors; makeup just makes me feel better.
In this comfortable position I set to the task at a leisurely pace.

ANXIETY

Anxiety hovers as I sit gazing out the front window, waiting for *the* phone call. Today was blood letting day to see if my poor little body is fit for another dose of toxins.
Message received:
'Your treatment will be delayed due to low ANC'.
Sigh... Better luck next week.
Absolute Neutrophil Count

INTOLERABLE

Tick - tick - tick ...
The clock is moving slowly now the end is so near.
Tick - tick - tick ...
My stomach churns. Tears prickle where once my eyelashes grew thickly.
Tick - tick - tick ...
Each sunrise brings another day that is not the one I'm waiting for. Last chemo is four long days ahead.
I hate waiting games.
Tick - tick - tick ...

HOW LUCKY I AM

Breast cancer care in my area is phenomenal. There have been no delays in getting the ball rolling from the day I first visited my GP. I have never felt abandoned, always knowing there is a friendly voice on the other end of the phone waiting to help. However...

IF ONLY THEY KNEW

How can I write this without sounding like I'm complaining? I'm not. Staff treating cancer patients should *know* how it feels, without having to suffer the illness. If they knew, they'd appreciate the tiny things that would make huge differences, like remembering to make that reassuring phone call as promised.

ON TENTERHOOKS

Tomorrow is my final chemo – I think. I've already had one delay so I'm sure it's OK, but I'll feel settled when I get the phone call to give me my 100% reassurance. Thank goodness I arranged for the nurse to ring no matter the result; the waiting is unbearable.

I AM DEVASTATED

It's 8pm and I am a wreck. Not much chance of a reassuring phone call now. She promised she'd ring. I specifically asked, saying I'd only ring her next morning so could she please put me out of my misery and ring whatever the result.
'Yes, of course I can.'

THE 'DAMN' BURSTS

I haven't cried many tears the last months. Tonight I make up for lost time. I feel sick with anxiety; I don't know what to do with myself. *Damn it!* I'm alone in the house and I yield to desperate tears. It's one of the worst nights of my life.

DO IT YOURSELF

I ring at 8:30am next morning and speak to nurse in question.
'No blood results yet, I'll have to ring you back.'
How dare the blood clinic hold onto my results for so long! They've had my blood for 24 hours.

She could've rung to tell me this last night.

FINAL CHEMO

I told the nurse that I was gutted the previous night re: lack of contact. Without honest feedback how will they ever know? I got a tissue for my tears but wasn't convinced she appreciated the validity of my feelings. Shame. How to make them understand? I wish I knew.

TOLERABLE

I believe positive thinking encourages philosophical attitude which in turn makes life tolerable.
A common question regarding chemotherapy:
'Is it horrific?'
'No. It's not nice, but not nearly as bad as I thought it would be.'
It could've been so much worse; I got off lightly with symptoms I experienced.

HERE AT LAST

The last four months all I have looked forward to is one less chemo treatment. Each visit was ticked off and I watched the list of six treatments grow shorter. Now it's done. I should feel elated but I don't. Instead, I feel anxious as I anticipate another aggressive therapy.

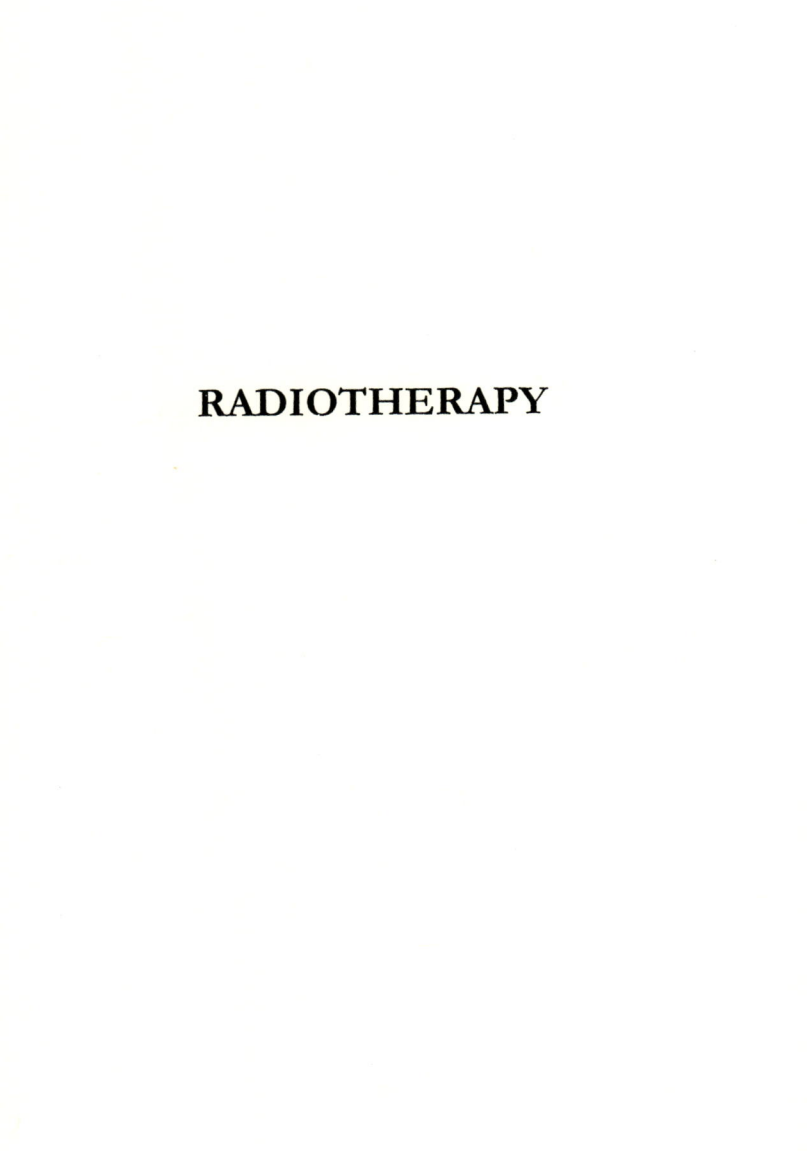

RADIOTHERAPY

MOVING RIGHT ALONG

Chemotherapy is like a traffic jam – delays – takes a long time to reach your destination.
Radiotherapy is like taking a diversion – longer than the shortest distance route – but because you keep on the move you feel you're progressing, and before you know it, the journey is over. Thank the Lord!

ANOTHER DRIVE TO HOSPITAL

My husband drives me to yet another hospital appointment. He's taken me to the appointments that mark beginnings; biopsy clinic, surgery, post op, first oncology visit and now we are nearing the end of the 'firsts' with regards to treatments. It's a shame knowing this doesn't make it any easier.

RADIOTHERAPY PLANNING SESSION

After all I've been through this should be easy. But tears threaten as the minutes tick by while I sit waiting for yet another appointment. Planning session for radiotherapy is imminent - unknown territory. It's got to be easier than chemo.

I've had enough. I want it to be over now.

ON THE TABLE

I am led to the radiation room.

STAFF AND PATIENTS ONLY BEYOND THIS POINT

I don't like being eligible to go beyond that point.
Strip to waist, get onto table, put hands in cuffs and three men scrutinize my breast for accurate measurement.
I would like to be somewhere else.

PIECE OF CAKE

I am finding it hard to keep it together at this appointment. I'm not feeling optimistic about entering another unknown zone of aggressive therapy. Silent tears flow and I can't find the plug. The doctor assures me radiotherapy is a 'piece of cake' compared to chemotherapy. I hope that's true.

BEYOND MY COMPREHENSION

You've seen hundreds of people in this situation, but to me, it's a new experience. You cannot know the emotional depths that cancer reaches if you haven't walked this path yourself. So please, forgive me if I'm unresponsive when you tell me that the next phase is easy in comparison.

TRANSPORT

When I first heard I'd need a minimum of 15 sessions of radiotherapy, strangely, my first thought was:
I don't want to do this alone and 15 lifts is a lot of favours to ask.
Offers of help were plentiful. I learned how to accept unconditionally. I was never alone.

PATIENTS

I think of my breasts as patients now rather than breasts. It makes it easier to enter the room where three people await my arrival, often one is male. I strip to the waist, climb onto the table and they inspect my breasts to make sure my position is perfect.

MIND OVER MATTER

I took a number of measures to protect myself from unwelcome radiation effects; homoeopathic *radiation remedy*, aloe vera gel, positive thinking, qigong, rest. When I read that cooling, moonlit visualisations could help prevent radiation burns, I added this to my list of preventative measures. Thankfully, my efforts have been worthwhile.

MOONLIT DIP

I am naked as I step into the cool lagoon on a clear moonlit night. I follow the path of the moon's reflection as I float on my back admiring the starry night sky.
This is where I go in my mind as I lie 'very still' during radiation treatments.

CUFFED

Torture chamber or kinky – I can't decide which best describes the position I lie in for radiation treatments. Don't fancy either description but they are what come to mind. I share my thought with staff. You've got to have a laugh; life can be too overwhelming without a good laugh.

TWILIGHT ZONE

Bandages removed from woman's face; she screams at mirror image. Pig faced doctors commiserate; one of 'her kind' takes her away. Remember that one? I feel like I'm entering a zone of 'my kind' as I cross hospital threshold. Inside I'll join others with minimal hair waiting for their appointments

CHATTY KATHY

LA3 delayed 30 minutes. The note goes up as I sit waiting for treatment; five minutes later they call me.
'That didn't seem a long wait' I say conversationally.
'Don't know why they put your file on top. Sorry you'll have to go back'
Tomorrow I'll speak not a word!

TRUE TO MY WORD

LA3 delayed 30 minutes. The note goes up again as I sit waiting for treatment; again, five minutes later they call my name.
'They've put your file before this gentleman, don't know why'.
I smile demurely and speak not a word as I follow obediently and enter the treatment room.

FINALLY

I've been looking forward to this day since December; seven long months. Today is the last day of my treatments. Though I resisted the need for treatments, I became accustomed to the routine. Now, oddly, as I await my final appointment time to arrive, I feel tearful. Utter relief I suspect.

LIBERATION

I feel now that I truly know the meaning of liberation. These last seven months my focus has been surviving hospital treatments. I have been so looking forward to looking forward to something other than one less treatment. And now treatments are complete I am loving the feeling of freedom.

POST TREATMENTS

FIRST FOLLOW UP

I enter feeling free as a bird, no more treatments – done. Nurse reels off instructions re: health awareness; when and who to phone for help. It was like being in a game of Snakes and Ladders and I slid down a snake to the feelings of my initial pre-chemo appointment.

BEING REALISTIC

Follow up appointment was a good reminder not to be complacent. I just feel I have had no time to celebrate the end of a long hard slog. The cancer ball keeps rolling downhill at a fast pace. End of long hard slog maybe, but not an absolute end. Bother!

REALITY

I guess I should be aware, now the pace is slowing, that the reality of my cancer might at last sink in. I was in shock from diagnosis to post-surgery; in fighting mode throughout therapies, determined to stay on top of the situation. Now there will be time to ponder.

I HAVE CHEMOTHERAPY

I've never really grasped the reality of my cancer. Throughout this journey I've felt that I've had chemotherapy rather than cancer. Chemotherapy was the biggest stumbling block for me. I found surgery straightforward; radiotherapy comparatively easy. Chemo had most difficult physical effects and by far the most dramatic emotional effect.

THAT'S JUST THE WAY IT IS TODAY

Today I feel sensitive and insecure; no particular reason. I feel cheesed off that I am still reliant on help and that this is no longer obvious now I'm getting back to normal, so I have to ask. Today I'm in a mood. I'm feeling irrational – so mind your backs!

ANXIOUS

I feel anxious when doctor appointments are looming. I have seldom needed medical assistance. These appointments bring my cancer forward and place it on the table where I am forced to look it straight in the eye. I prefer keeping it at the back of the cupboard of my mind.

ANOTHER FOLLOW UP

It's been 11 months since I've seen the surgeon. I'm conscious that I will be a file, a hospital number, a scar he will recognize as his own work; but I won't be me, Kathy. I'll be Kathleen. I know I can't expect anything more but it troubles me nonetheless.

NO NEED TO WORRY

Drugs and knowledge have equal healing status in my book; drugs for physical symptoms, knowledge for stabilising emotional health.
My surgeon and my oncologist are my kind of doctors. They answer my barrage of questions in a patient and non-condescending manner. I must re-read this when next appointment looms!

HAIR

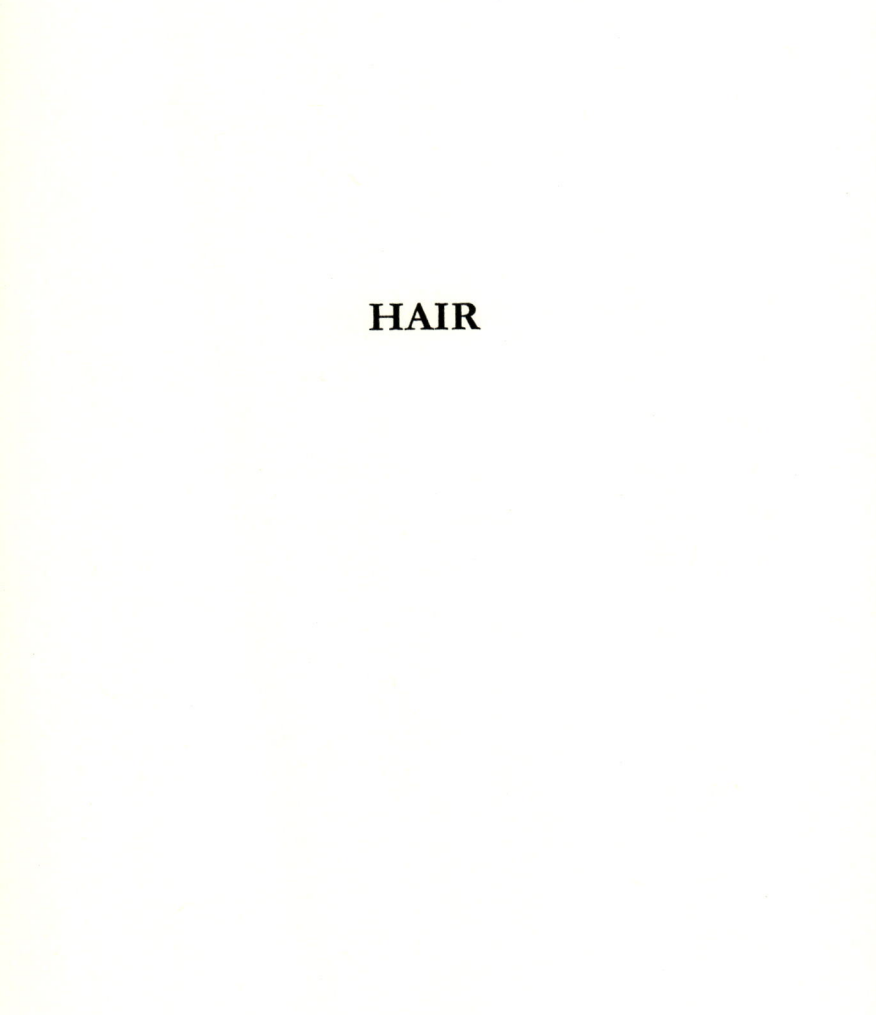

DECISIONS

I've made an appointment to have my hair permed. That was before lump; before biopsy. Now I await diagnosis and wonder if I should cancel. Perm won't last long if chemo reckons in the equation.
No, I will not be pessimistic. I'll have the perm and hope for the best.

THERE IT GOES

Preparations have been made. I've had my hair cut shorter than it's ever been – I like it, it suits me.
Day 16 after first chemo treatment and my scalp begins to feel very irritating, itchy and sore. I give it a scratch and my hands come away full of hair.

TAKE IT AWAY

Hair lasts two days before Eddie shaves my head. I can't bear to watch it fall out daily.

My brave son sets about my head with a #3 clipper; not short enough, #1 next day; uncomfortably prickly, electric shaver next and finally razor. At last, a smooth pate – how bizarre!

I KEEP FORGETTING

I roam the house bareheaded in the evenings. I'm getting used to the idea of being bald. As time passes my lack of hair is not a major concern. When I pass a mirror and catch sight of my image it surprises me. *'Bloody hell, I forgot I was bald!'*

A SHADOW OF MY FORMER SELF

The strangest thing about being bald is seeing my shadow when I'm doing qigong by candlelight; so striking with the clear cut shape of my head. It surprises me every time I see it. It's almost stranger than my mirror image. Funny how things strike you differently than you imagined they might.

WIG

I had met cancer patients wearing wigs and was often surprised that it wasn't natural hair.
I wasn't sure about wearing a wig but I got one just in case. Natural as it looked, I felt more natural wearing scarves. Wearing the wig made me feel depressed; I felt untruthful.

SCARVES

I thought I'd probably wear scarves once my hair disappeared. I had three lovely squares I used as neck scarves. I practised winding them round my head when I still had hair. Two had a fringe – pretend hair! I quite liked the look – 'aging hippy' suits me nicely.

NO MORE BAD HAIR DAYS!

One thing about being bald, you never have a bad hair day! I don't have bad wig days because, as attractive as my wig is, I can't bring myself to wear it. I have bad eyebrow days. Sometimes it takes ages to get eyebrows just the right shade and shape.

RAISED EYEBROWS

'Well at least you haven't lost your eyebrows'.
This is the most common comment from people who see me for the first time since chemotherapy began.
'Yes I have. I'm a good artist with an excellent eyebrow pencil'.
They have a closer look and say, 'It *is* good isn't it?'

NOT A HAIR OUT OF PLACE

Not a hair at all. It continued to grow after ritual shaving but remained weak. When my body was finally freed of drugs it began growing strong. Downy white fuzz became thicker and darker; my bare scalp began to disappear. And this morning, there was a hair out of place!

DAILY HAIR REPORT

My husband gets a daily hair report……
'Feel that, I feel like a little chick.'
'When I shampooed my hair this morning there was lather!'
'Look at that one sticking out; I need to comb that down now!'
'Ann bought me a baby brush, now I can brush my hair.'

IT HAS TO BE FOR ME

The prospect of losing my hair didn't worry me; there were too many other concerns to consider. My choice in dealing with my baldness had to be what made me comfortable. The wig was a no-goer from the start. Now my hair begins to grow the scarf is abandoned.

YOU BET!

On seeing my hair for the first time he asked, 'You going out like that?'

'You bet. I've decided I'm ready to face the world and if the world isn't ready for me they'll just have to get over it because I'm in control of this situation.'

'Good for you.'

MANIKINS

I tell my 23 year old son I'm ready to go out without my scarf on. My hair is growing back nicely now chemo is finished.

'No, don't', he says. 'People will think you are an escaped manikin and they will pick you up and return you to the store.'!!

GROWING CONCERN

Had you sported a bald pate you'd appreciate the signs: the invisible fuzz; the pigment making an appearance. You wouldn't look at me seeing my minimal hair as the Scarlet Letter it is, screaming CANCER PATIENT.
If it makes you uncomfortable, don't look at my head. Look at my smile.

IN A WORD

My first walk in public with minimal hair was to the post box. The only person I encountered had less hair than me! Next walk to post box a toddler only capable of minimal words was walking with her dad and when she saw me she pointed and said, 'haircut'.

IS THERE ANYONE OUT THERE WATCHING?

Yesterday I went out alone and scarf-less for the first time. In the local shop I watched people as I walked down the aisles, looking to see if anyone was checking out my minimal hair. Surprisingly, they weren't. I'm comfortable with this temporary look now, so it doesn't matter anyway.

YOU CAN'T THROW A BATHROBE ON YOUR EYEBROWS

The postman rings the doorbell. Bother. I have just stepped out of the shower.
'Eddie, will you please go down, I'm not presentable.'
I thought I'd be able to cope with answering the door with limited head hair, (1/2" long now!), but I am *not* facing anyone with no eyebrows!

ANOTHER FIRST

I did it. I walked into that room full of people I sing with, head with minimal hair held high, and they gave me a round of applause! I invited all to pat my fuzzy head at break time and many did. I do hang out with a nice crowd.

CHOP AND CHANGE

Sometimes when I look in the mirror I'm delighted to see the progress of my hair growth. Other times when I look in the mirror I feel tearful to see my skinhead look. It reminds me that I have had to endure a battle with an uninvited and unwelcome disease.

GREETINGS

My body has been free of chemo drugs for eight weeks and I can now run my fingers through my lovely soft hair.
I bought myself a card in honour of my returning hair - it bears a small sketch of a rear view of a toddler brushing her hair.

IT ALL DEPENDS ON HOW YOU LOOK AT IT

When my son shaved my head with the #3 comb it looked shockingly short. That's when I started covering my head.　Now my hair has re-grown to that length it looks positively long to me; a welcome change from being bald.　Nothing could persuade me to cover my head now.

WELCOME BACK

I love the way my hair feels. It is just long enough for me to run my fingers through, and I often do. It is dense and strong and soft. The colour is lighter than before but there is still a hint of the original red tinge. Welcome back hair.

14 WEEKS POST CHEMO

My 'no hair days' are over.
My 'bad hair days' are coming.
But just for now I am going to wallow in the luxury of simply having 'hair days'.
I love, love, LOVE my hair.
It may be short,
but it's soft,
and it's not white (phew),
and it's THERE!

CONVERSELY

I told my family today that I don't know if I'll be able to cope with having hair! I'm so used to this short style. I thought the gradual growth would grow on me (so to speak) but, interesting as it is to observe, it's peculiar dealing with hair again.

17 WEEKS POST CHEMO

14 weeks hair growth

During tonight's hair inspection I see there are little curly waves hugging the back of my head. Well, well, I think I will end up with a curly bonce. That will save on hairdresser fees! But I don't usually have tight curls. Might have to return to this short style.

NEW SHADOW

All of a sudden today the curls have reached the top of my head. And so – my shadow no longer looks bald! There are little spiky bits breaking up that smooth round shadow. Thank goodness for that. I've been waiting long enough for this little breakthrough in my 'hair history'!

HAIRCUT

Big day today, I have an appointment with the hairdresser! This day seemed a long way off not many weeks ago. When I rang to make an appointment she asked if I wanted a shampoo.
"Yes please."
It's such a novelty to need a shampoo. I'm going to enjoy this.

BACK TO NORMAL

I have arrived at the hairdressers for my first post chemo haircut.
I've had my shampoo, (lovely), and I am sitting in the hairdresser's chair facing the mirror. He combs through my wet hair as if this is normal, yet I feel I am going through a rite of passage.

NEW LOOK

Thanks to chemotherapy I now have the hair style I've always been too chicken to try – extremely short. And now it's here, with the bonus of curls, I see I was right in thinking it is the look for me. Drastic way to find a look that suits!

BREASTS

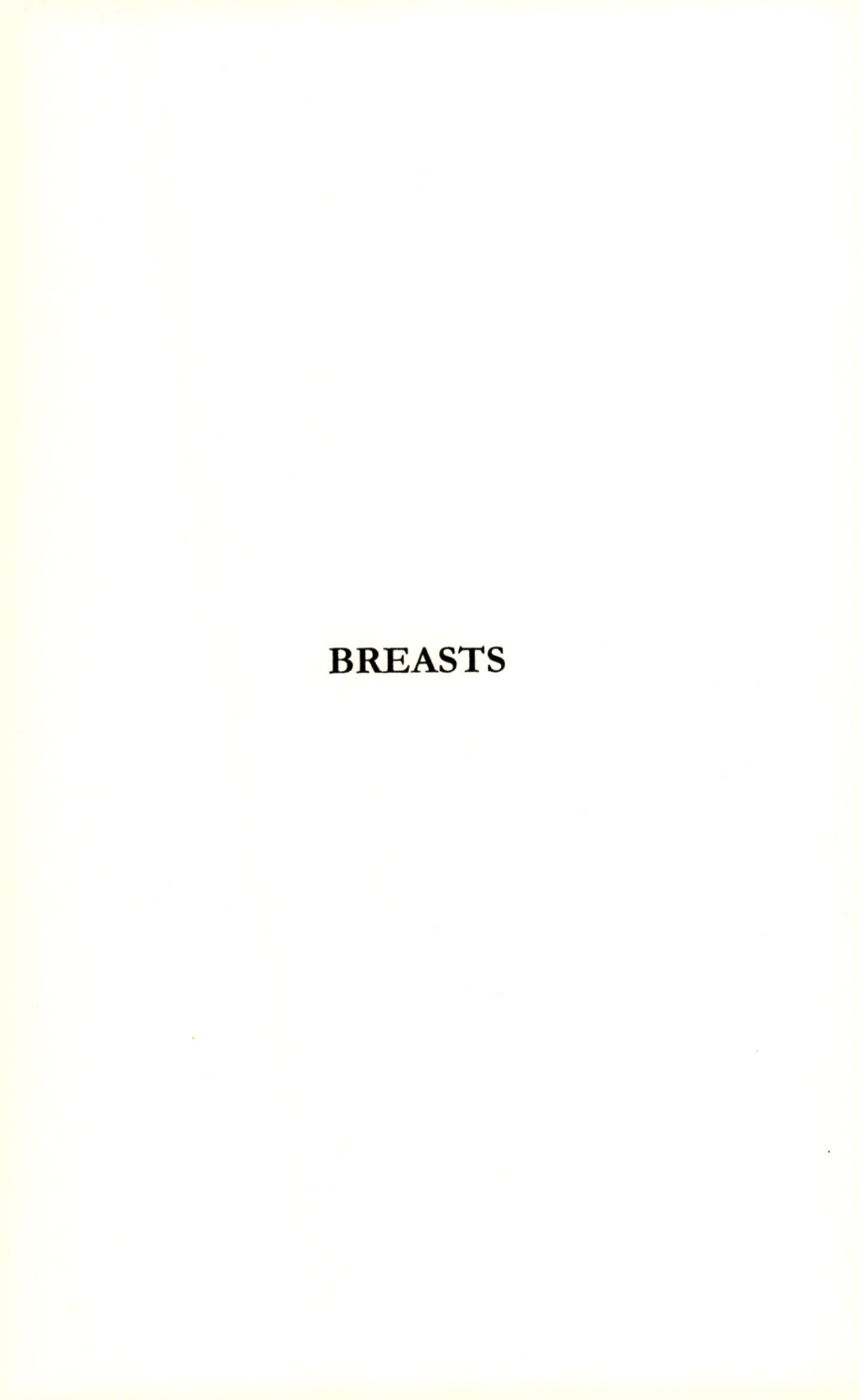

EVERY DAY

Not once a month, everyday. Check your breasts everyday so you never forget. Stand in front of the mirror when dressing every morning and admire your breasts as you check for visual discrepancies, feel for telltale lumps. If there's something amiss, best to find it early; if not, praise God.

INTIMATE TERMS

I'm on intimate terms with my left breast. Each night, since I discovered my lump, I've had a nightly breast inspection. My poor little breast has been through the wars; aubergine-like after surgery, reddened scar, weeping wound, stitch poking through, the brown tinge stubbornly remains and now the radiation blush.

SHY NO MORE

I have always been shy of my breasts. I remember a painfully embarrassing doctor appointment when I was a pre-teen where paediatrician and my mother commented on my budding breasts. The memory makes me cringe even now. However, after seven months of breast cancer treatment, I am shy no more!

SELF CONFIDENCE

I'm thankful that my self confidence remains in tact in spite of this brush with cancer. I have no worries about my scarring. I don't feel less of a woman. I feel I am a more powerful woman; I have survived the experience. Been there, done that and moving on.

FRIENDS

A TROUBLE SHARED

I have proved to myself that *a trouble shared is a trouble halved.* I shared my trouble with so many people that it became fragmented into tiny pieces. Whenever I was troubled there was always someone there to help me cope. Sharing helped me to bear this very heavy load.

SMOOTHER ROAD AHEAD

All the cards I have received throughout this seven month journey cover both sides of my kitchen door. I have kept them there for moral support and they have been a great comfort as I walked this rocky path. I envision a clear door soon leading to a smoother walkway.

__SISTERS__

Thank God for the immediacy of email. Email is a lifeline.
Email makes my sister, who lives 6000 miles away, seem like she's next door. She has been an angel to me throughout this challenging time in my life. I can tell her anything and there's always a supportive reply.

__CANCER BUDDY__

She rings me three times a week to make sure I'm OK. I call her my telephone babysitter. She listens to my cancer chat, tells me her news and we put the world to rights:
Did you see that TV programme; hear that news …
What a good cancer buddy.

VALIDATION

'Am I making a big deal out of this? Some days it's hard to know, I feel like I should hurt or something.'
'Yes, it's a huge deal' my friend reassures me.
I need this validation. I need to know that today's feelings are OK and tomorrow's will be too.

BROAD SHOULDERS

My email contacts have borne broad shoulders throughout my therapies. It's easy to spill your feelings, share your raw emotions, via cyberspace. I'm afraid I've been guilty of wallowing on occasion and I thank my many communicants for bearing with me. They've played a large part in my healing process.

HOW ARE YOU TODAY?

How am I today? It depends who's asking…
"Coping better than I expected I would"
"Lacking energy, but very well considering"
"I've been spending time with my 'best friend' (TV) like my sister told me to"
"I'm pissed off - so if you don't really want to know, hang up now!"

SPEAKING OF FRIENDS.

Since beginning chemo, makeup has become one of my very best friends. I felt so exposed when I lost my hair that I felt I had to make a feature of my face to take the attention away from that lack of hair, especially my lack of eyebrows and eyelashes.

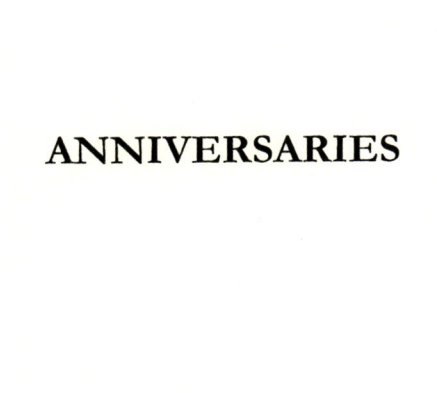

ANNIVERSARIES

WHO KNOWS WHEN THOSE TEARS WILL HIT

I can be chatting quite happily and BAM; my lip quivers, my throat tightens, my eyes moisten and I'm rendered speechless; it's a real struggle to fight off the tears. At present I seem to be living a battery of 'anniversary' feelings. Last year was full of unknowns. Now - I know …

TELL ME IT'S NOT TRUE

I love the song of this title from *Blood Brothers*. It's always made me cry when I've listened to it. Now, as November 19th looms, it springs to mind.
"Tell me it's not true. Say it's just a story. Say it's just a show on the radio…"
If only.

ANNIVERSARY

This coming Saturday is November 19th. It will be one year since I found my lump. A year since the anxiety of cancer entered my life. I don't dwell on it, but when I'm alone with my thoughts, tears prickle whilst that original feeling of dread replays in my mind

CELEBRATE

When my friend is visiting we always make a beeline for our favourite shopping mall.
I feel better about shopping if I make excuses for the splurge. In August we celebrated my end of treatments.
She's here again, and off we go. Today we celebrate my cancer anniversary in style!

BALLET

When Pete suggested we book for the Birmingham ballet early December, my heart froze. I was back in the car December 3rd 2004 with the radiologist's prediction of cancer ringing in my ears - heading home instead of to the ballet.
'Oh. Yes. Ok then'.
This anniversary is dampening my enthusiasm.

DEEP DOWN

I feel as if there is a sob in the deepest part of my being begging to be set free. The tears that appear unexpectedly are the tip of the rumble waiting to erupt. I think it's this challenging year coming to an end. But I don't sob; I reflect.

THE LAST DAY

New Year's Eve 2005

I say I will be glad to see the back of 2005; that I welcome a new, cancer free year. Of course I welcome a cancer free year. But many good things happened in 2005 as well and I mustn't let the memory of cancer therapies overshadow these pleasant memories.

SAME 'OL, SAME 'OL

New Year's Day

I discovered today that my 'just bear with me' moments are still with me. I met someone I hadn't seen in years and when the conversation turned to last year's cancer experience, (as it inevitably does), unexpected tears began to flow. Maybe I'll get used to the unexpected one day.

GENERALLY SPEAKING

TIME PASSES

19/11   Lump detected
22/11   GP appointment
24/11   Clinic appointment received
3/12   Biopsy clinic
9/12   Results
21/12   Surgery
30/12   Lab results
11/01   Oncologist
16/02   Chemo begins
15/06   Chemo ends
6/07   Radiotherapy begins
26/07   Radiotherapy ends
HURRAH!!!

A time warp has made this time creep past, yet, whiz by.

JUST BEAR WITH ME

Every phone call I made the few weeks following my diagnosis began with this preamble:
'Just bear with me, I can't say this without crying'.
I'd pause, gather strength,
'I've been diagnosed with breast cancer ...'
There have been a few 'Just bear with me' situations these last few months.

CHILDLIKE

I have reverted to a childlike state in that I need constant reassurance. I need to know exactly what will happen, how long I'm likely to be waiting, what's involved in treatment regimes. I need to be told I'm coping well. And I'm grateful when I'm indulged in these needs.

WAITING IS THE WORST PART

I have waited for:
Initial doctor appointment
Clinic appointment card
Clinic appointment
Doctors to see me
Surgery date
Surgery
Start of chemo
Go ahead for chemo after blood tests
Each chemo appointment
Radiation appointments
End of treatments

I will never, *ever* get used to the anxiety that accompanies such waiting.

STATISTICS

- 30% of female cancers are breast cancer
- Four out of five cases of breast cancer involve women aged over 50
- Most cases have no family history of the disease
- 90% of cases are discovered by selves
- The majority of cases involve the left breast

That pretty much sums me up.

RECORD NUMBER

In the 15 years previous to my cancer diagnosis, visits to my doctor were mainly for routine tests. Since cancer, beginning 14 months ago, I've had a record 62 appointments with medical professionals! It's wonderful that this amount of care is available, but incredible that I have needed such care.

MARKING TIME

Do you mark your existence by landmarks in your life? For example: when you were still in school, when you still lived in parental home, before marriage, before children ...

I have some new ones to add to my current repertoire: Before lump, before cancer, pre-chemo, when I still had hair...

ROCKY ROAD

Finding the lump landed me on the cliff edge. Diagnosis caused me to lose my footing. Surgery made me send for the troops. Chemotherapy made me glad I'd sent for the troops. Radiotherapy, being so near the end of treatments, allowed a glimmer of light showing a road less rocky.

BAD ATTITUDE

One of the characters from my favourite TV medical dramas described his brain tumour thus:
'My tumour was just a bunch of cells with bad attitude.'
I'm going to adopt that way of thinking. My bad attitude tumour has been overcome by medical treatment and my good attitude. Good riddance.

POORLY?

I've never considered myself sick or poorly throughout my cancer journey. Mostly I've been emotionally challenged. I'm glad my gut reaction was to share the news with everyone I know. Support received as a result gave me the courage to tackle cancer head on. Poorly? Not me. I'm fighting fit.

IS THERE ANYTHING GOOD YOU CAN SAY ABOUT CANCER?

Yes, there is actually. Before cancer I had no first hand experience of the power of prayer. Because of cancer I've been in a position of need and I've had the honour of being on the receiving end of family, friends and acquaintances filling that need. And ... I've lost weight!

MY NEW CHOICE OF DIET

I avoid red meat, dairy products, caffeine and alcohol. I consume fresh fruit, vegetables, (lots of orange ones), grains, pulses, nuts, seeds and soya products, preferably organic; some fish and occasionally eggs.

I've lost unwelcome weight; remained in good health throughout cancer therapies, and good health continues.

Good job Kathy!

WATER

At my radiotherapy planning session I was told I should drink 2.5 litres of water per day during treatment time. I was already managing 2 litres per day and had drunk 3 litres on some chemo days. Water is one of many things to which I credit my good health.

CHANGE OF DIET

I'm often asked if I'll continue with my diet. Why would I change my diet when my cancer treatments are complete? I'd regain the stone I was so pleased to lose, I would be less healthy and I would not enjoy my food nearly as much as I do now.

ANTIPERSPIRANTS

I've read that parabens in antiperspirants can contribute to breast cancer. There are two schools of thought on this claim. There is no concrete scientific proof that this is so, though some agree further studies are necessary. Meanwhile, I will use paraben free products to be on the safe side.

PARABENS AND PESTICIDES

If parabens are a possible link to breast cancer, why are they in most cosmetics available for purchase?
Why are we penalised by having to pay high prices for organic food when pesticides are clearly hazardous to our health?
Why are these hazardous chemicals forced upon us everywhere we shop?

IT'S MY CANCER AND I'LL CRY IF I WANT TO

My mission in life now is to help people understand that it's OK if someone cries.

DON'T PANIC. It's an honest reaction that needs expressing, that's all.

It's about the other person, not you.

Don't get embarrassed; don't feel you need to make it better. Just go with the flow.

TEARS

Sometimes memories of particular events promote tears. No matter how well you have healed with regard to that event, the mention of it feels the same as the first occurrence. Like when I received my first invitation for a breast screening mammogram a month after my breast cancer treatments ended…

I'M AFRAID OF NOT KNOWING

I think what I'm most afraid of is, not knowing. Not knowing where my cancer came from; not knowing whether or not it will return. I'm afraid of not knowing to what extent cancer has affected me physically.
I reckon 'not knowing' is one of the scariest things about life.

TALK TO ME

For me, the fear of being treated like a patient rather than an ordinary person, or being avoided because someone is at a loss for words, is as big as the fear of cancer itself. Let's talk Cancer. If it's out in the open, it becomes a bit less scary.

CANCER SURVIVOR

If I'm a cancer survivor that means I've had cancer. Because everything was dealt with so promptly I haven't got used to that in spite of all I've been through. So when it was said today,
"There is a survivor amongst us"
I cried tears of sadness; tears of pride.

AND FURTHERMORE…

When it was said today,
"There is a survivor amongst us"
I felt very similar to the way I felt when the consultant said,
"We've had the result of your biopsy and it has come back positive for cancer."
It felt surreal. I felt like this shouldn't apply to me.

WHAT'S IN A WORD?

I am not *sick;* I am dealing with a *health issue*
I am not a cancer *victim;* I am a cancer *patient*
I am not *struggling* with cancer; I am *battling* cancer
Don't offer me your *sympathy;* Offer me your *support*
Cancer is not in *control;* I am *in charge*

AFFIRMATION

It's not what happens,
But how I respond to what happens
That determines the quality of my life

I'd repeated this affirmation so often by the time cancer came knocking at my door that this had become an automatic response to stress.

It's proved a good rule to live by.

CROSSROADS

I feel I'm at a crossroads regarding my feelings about my cancer. It's fast becoming past tense yet I seem to want to hang on to it.

I don't want to become complacent because I'm afraid of having to learn the lesson all over again if I let it go.

I WISH

I have to believe that chemotherapy has rid my body of all stray cancer cells; that radiotherapy has removed the possibility of cancer returning. I know this isn't set in stone, but I have to believe this to make what I've gone through worthwhile.

I wish – long life to me!

PATCHWORK

Cancer is a big patch in the patchwork of my life. This patch may look rough on the outside, but gold flecks catch the light; love, prayers, pathways to a healthier lifestyle; new friendships, closer bonds within relationships. I cannot deny these golden threads cancer has woven into my life.

THANK YOU GOD FOR EVERYTHING

I have a lot to be thankful for, supportive family and friends, positive attitude, little stress in my life and not least, my good health. If cancer presents itself in one's life, best to be in good shape and present as a strong warrior – God knows it's a tough battle.

IF YOU OR ANYONE YOU LOVE HAS CANCER…

I wish for you the strength to deal with it positively. I hope you'll be able to recognise the angels in your life and let them help you cope; that you're able to accept this unwelcome visitor and that you hang on to as much control as you are able.

ABOUT THE AUTHOR

Kathy is a native Californian residing in England where she lives with her husband and two sons. After being involved with early years education for fourteen years she changed careers and is now a practising Reflexologist. The format of this journal of 50 word thoughts was inspired by an exercise assigned in a writing class.

Printed in the United Kingdom
by Lightning Source UK Ltd.
112375UKS00001B/106-120